Yoga

Thorsons First Directions

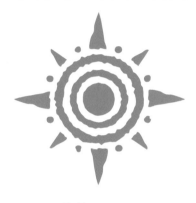

Yoga
Cheryl Isaacson

Thorsons
An Imprint of HarperCollins*Publishers*
77-85 Fulham Palace Road,
Hammersmith, London W6 8JB

The Thorsons website address is:
www.thorsons.com

Published by Thorsons 2001

10 9 8 7 6 5 4 3 2 1

Text derived from *Principles of Yoga* published by Thorsons 1996

Editor: Louise McNamara
Design: Wheelhouse Creative Ltd.
Production: Melanie Vandevelde
Photography by Henry Allen and PhotoDisk Europe

A catalogue record for this book is available from the British Library

ISBN 0 00711038 3

Printed and bound in Hong Kong.

Contents

Yoga

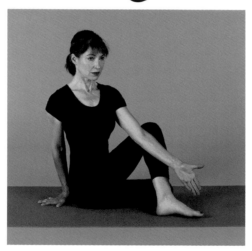

is a time-honoured system of balancing

mind, body and spirit

What is Yoga?

Not just knots ...

What do you think of when someone mentions yoga? People bending and stretching, balancing and twisting, in the classic poses now familiar to the health scene? Deep relaxation and mind control? Chanting and meditating and staring into candle flames? If so, then you are right on all counts – but you are only seeing part of the whole. The practices that we call 'yoga' today are just one small part of what is actually a many sided, practical, life-enhancing discipline.

Yoga was originally part of the mystical wisdom of Indian philosophy, but today we mostly concentrate on the body postures, or asanas, with perhaps some breath control and a little meditation thrown in. The postures certainly help you to become fit and supple, but they are only one aspect of the complete way of life that yoga can bring.

Yoga also offers:
- practical techniques for living life healthily and holistically, from following the correct diet to deep breathing and body strengthening
- a complete code of ethics for daily life
- simple methods for relaxing and meditating
- postures for a toned, supple, healthy, strong body
- tried and tested ways to find profound personal peace and stability.

Yoga can affect your whole life and there are many different ways of applying it. It is not just for the young and fit, and – most importantly – you can start at any time. Yoga has something for a truly wide range of people, whatever the state of their mind and body.

Yoga's spiritual path

The desire for spiritual experience has led many to look to the religious systems of the East. Yoga is, at heart, a spiritual path that offers powerful rituals and meditation techniques to help us enter other states of consciousness. People call this many different things: a spiritual sense, a connection with a greater power, a higher consciousness, even God. Whatever form it takes, it seems to be as important to human satisfaction now as it was 3,000 years ago.

Mystics and sages show us that spiritual bliss and extraordinary peace is possible. However, the closest most of us get to this is a flash of feeling extraordinarily peaceful and 'at one with the universe'. While this feeling may not last, it does open us up to a different state of being. If you want to achieve some peace of mind, or connect with a more spiritual part of yourself, then this is possible through yoga.

Yoga is the mystical religious philosophy of India.

Creating balance

Yoga creates a sense of balance – from offering practical advice on following the right diet to allowing you to calm the mind by consciously detaching from the stresses of everyday life. Even though it is thousands of years old, yoga can work wonders in present times.

Yoga's philosophical path

The ideas behind yoga are very closely linked to Indian philosophy. This is made up of many highly complex ideas, which are so much part of India's hugely diverse religious tradition that the two are inseparable. There are six main branches of Indian philosophy and yoga is one of these branches. Yoga represents the mystical tradition, and aims to bring about a union between the individual being and the universal consciousness. In fact, the word 'yoga' is most commonly translated as 'union'.

The Origins of Yoga

Some forms of yoga can be traced back 2,500 years, while others are said to be medieval. Physical, or Hatha yoga, probably dates from around the tenth century AD.

The Vedic Age

Between 1,800 BC and 1,000 BC the Indus Valley was inhabited by Sanskrit-speaking tribes known as the Vedic people. They give us our first firm links with yoga. Hymns dating from that time (such as the *Rig Veda* and the *Atharva-Veda*) describe practices which we would recognize as powerful meditations. In fact the origins of all the ideas that we think of as 'yogic' are here.

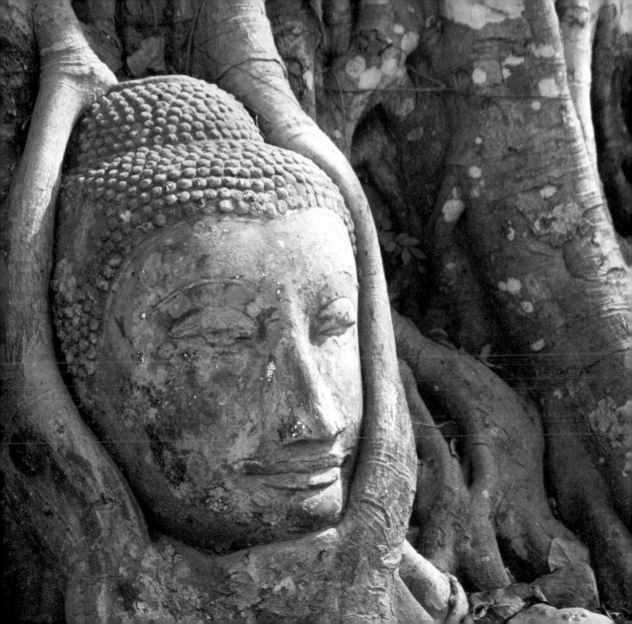

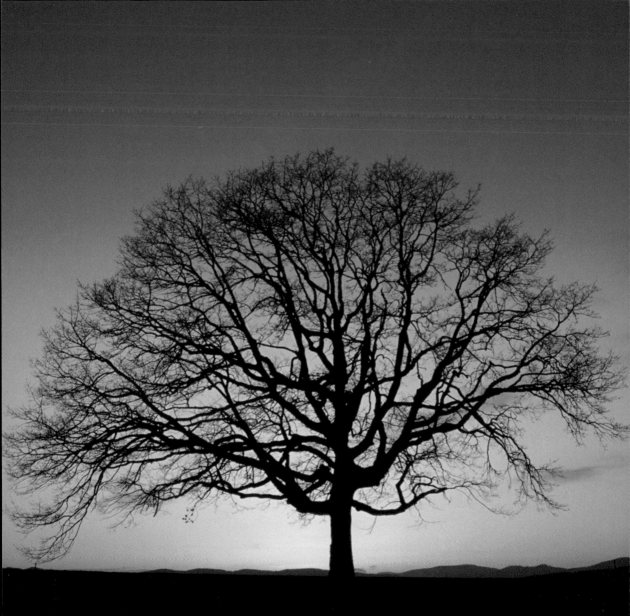

Terracotta seals have been found in the Indus valley, dating from around 3,000 years ago. These show figures, probably ancient gods, sitting in recognizably yogic postures, such as the famous lotus pose, with legs folded, hands on their knees and the feet crossed one on top of the other.

The Indian epics

The six main branches of Indian philosophy arose around 600–500 BC. Then, from about 8 BC a more mystical trend developed with the writing of yoga's most important literary works, the *Upanishads*. These describe developments within the whole Hindu culture, which was just beginning to form its own religious identity. Along with the *Upanishads*, the national epics of India, the *Ramayana* (5th or 6th century BC) and the *Mahabharata* (5th century BC), are important. The *Mahabharata* contains the *Bahagavad Gita*, a treatise that looks at the central yogic precept of non-attachment to material things. It also contains another section on yoga theory.

Yoga through the ages

These texts have been added to and developed through time, and through the ages yoga has embraced a great variety of teachings, writings and practices. The most famous person to expound on yoga from a philosophical point of view was Patanjali, who wrote the *Yoga Sutras* some time between 200 BC and 200 AD. He condensed yogic wisdom into a series of brief aphorisms on spiritual practice and power, still highly relevant today. With yoga, spiritual unity seemed to be accessible through anything from sexual bliss to total isolation. But the ultimate goal of all these practices was enlightenment.

Hatha yoga

Physical yoga, (usually called by its Sanskrit name, Hatha yoga), developed in the tenth century AD. Then, a legendary charismatic healer and celibate called Goraksha wrote a work called *Hatha-Yoga*. This became a standard text which was developed and added to until the mid-14th century, when *Hatha Yoga Pradipika*, the best known work of classical yoga practice, appeared. It describes the basic cleansing methods of the body, breath control methods, energy-controlling hand positions, and ways of holding the body to intensify life energy. It also goes through in detail the postures as we know them today.

In the 19th century Queen Victoria was very interested in yoga and would summon Indian sages to perform their strange body contortions.

The rise of modern yoga

Yoga really took off in the West after Swami Sivananda, one of the great Indian yoga practitioners, decided to spread yoga's message in the 1950s. The time was right – spiritual ideas were becoming fashionable, along with interest in self-development and the growth of health and body consciousness. Yoga was the ideal way to incorporate all these, and the 1960s and 1970s saw an enormous growth in the yoga 'industry'. Other modern masters who have influenced yoga in the west are BKS Iyengar, Desikachar and Pramahamsa Yogananda, who

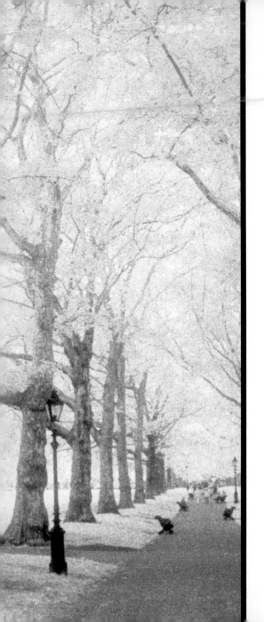

inspired many Westerners on the spiritual yogic path with his book, *Autobiography of a Yogi*.

Yoga today

Gone are the days when doing yoga meant dedicating your life to weird and wonderful practices or isolating yourself from family and friends. Today, the most separation from normal life that comes about is usually just an hour or so at a yoga class, once a week. But this is not to put down modern yoga teaching. Relaxation, peace of mind, health and fitness may be the main aims of the modern yoga student, but the age-old goals of connecting with a spiritual sense and broadening your consciousness are still very possible.

What Can Yoga Do For Me?

All the major systems of the body are influenced by regular Hatha yoga practice.

• It Stretches the Muscles ...
Yoga postures involve deep stretching movements – even muscles you didn't know you had are involved. But unlike other forms of exercise, the muscles are given a gentle, controlled stretch, without any strain, which means they can extend gradually and safely. And once your muscles gain flexibility, they become stronger and better-toned.

• It Delays the Ageing Process ...
Regular practice delays the ageing process by keeping muscles and ligaments moving. Although you may experience muscular aches and

pains after a yoga session, these will soon wear off, leaving you refreshed. Yoga should never leave you feeling jumpy or exhausted.

• It Loosens and Strengthens the Spine ...

As the muscles loosen and stretch, so do the ligaments which hold the spine in place. Instead of being held rigidly, the bones become free to move back into a more natural alignment. This is especially true of the spinal vertebrae, as many of the yoga postures work directly on the spinal column. The postures are also preventative, and help guard against slipped discs.

• It Improves Circulation ...

Your circulatory system improves through regular, deep breathing. With yoga you become more aware of your breath, and will start to use more of your lungs. Oxygenated blood is pumped more effectively to all the organs, revitalizing them and carrying away toxins. The inverted postures help blood circulation, reversing the blood flow, and also improve lymph drainage.

• It Helps Digestion ...

The digestive system is helped by the internal massaging action which some of the postures perform on the organs. Twisting postures, and those which involve the back bending forwards and backwards, will help stimulate the digestive organs. The improved circulatory process allows cleansing blood supply to reach the stomach and intestines.

• It Calms the Nerves ...

The nervous and endocrine systems are also affected. Yoga's concentration on the spine, through which the major nerve pathways flow, helps to control nervous energy. Regular yoga practice is well-known for reducing anxiety and panic states.

• It Balances Hormones and Emotions ...

Many people find that hormonal irregularities, such as menstrual problems, right themselves. Hyperactivity and lethargy can be overcome and emotions become more stable through doing yoga.

• And That's Not All ...

Anyone who practises long enough will soon find changes taking place which are quite subtle. They will begin to notice improvements in their health, energy and mental state, becoming calmer and more detached from the worries of daily life. They feel clearer, more directed and more purposeful.

• It Helps Cast Off Bad Habits ...

Yoga can also help you develop a growing awareness and sensitivity. Once your inner harmony starts to grow, bad habits are much easier to cast off. When you are more in touch with yourself, you no longer need to smoke, drink so much alcohol, or eat the things you know are bad for you. Yoga also helps you develop qualities such as discipline, patience and intelligence.

• And Finally ...

Yoga can give you a natural high, by helping you to tap into a higher consciousness. However, rather than this altered state being the temporary result of a substance you have taken, likely to let you down to normal reality with a bump, this state can stay with you. And, while drugs and other methods can cause us to become dangerously out of touch with normal reality, with yoga you will remain stable.

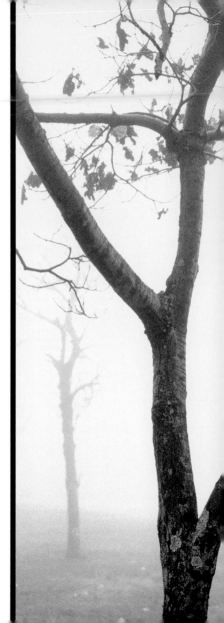

Finding a Teacher and Class

The many paths of yoga

The yoga we mostly practice today is Hatha, the yoga of physical posture. But just as there are all sorts of personalities and a whole variety of lifestyles, so there are different yogic paths to suit these. If you want to you can find teachers of yogas which emphasize the use of sound and chanting, of love and devotion, of the mind rather than the body. There is not space in this book to cover all these paths, but if you find that you are particularly attracted to one of these then follow up the contacts in the Resource Guide (*see page* 89). Whatever system you follow, you will gain a sense of the wholeness of yoga.

The different schools of yoga

Today you are likely to hear yoga systems referred to by the teachers who originated them, or to the specific practices associated with them. These schools have taken elements from the classical tradition and emphasized particular aspects. The most popular types include:

- **Iyengar Yoga**. BKS Iyengar developed this system, combining physical (Hatha) and mental yoga, which he believes are inter-dependent. Iyengar yoga is quite physically demanding, with great precision required for each posture. Once mastered, it offers a complete means of tuning body, mind and spirit.

- **Sivananda Yoga**. This system was devised by Swami Vishnu Devananda from the teachings of his master, Swami Sivananda. It includes smooth-running breathing practices and postures, and diet and positive thinking are also emphasized.

- **Astanga Vinyasa**. Often called 'power yoga', this is suitable for the very fit, who want their yoga to act as a strong physical work-out. The postures are performed fast and continuously, with sequences of movements, encouraging the build up of heat in the body and a strong flow of energy.

The yoga class – What to expect

Your first class will probably be a Hatha yoga class. This is the most physical path, and the most accessible. Hatha yoga should be done with the help of a properly trained teacher, at least initially. Don't be tempted to try to do too much too soon. Your class will probably consist of the well-known body postures, practised in a sequence which will differ according to your teacher. Generally, standing postures are performed first, then sitting postures, with relaxation at the end.

Breathing practices (*see page* 68), (called *pranayama* in Sanskrit), may also be a feature in your class. They help to cleanse your body, and much more besides. Breath is said to contain essential life force and how we take it in and use it is crucial.

The chakras

Your yoga teacher may talk about the chakras, and how the different postures can work on the different chakras, or energy points. The seven chakras are part of yoga philosophy; they are believed to be little vortices of energy, each with a different function:

- The root chakra is located at the perineum. It governs the lower limbs and the sense of smell, as well as the emotion of fear and the sense of security. It is associated with the colour red.
- The base chakra is located at the genitals. It governs sexuality and physical energy, the hands and the sense of taste. It is associated with the colour orange.
- The navel, or solar plexus chakra, is located at the base of the sternum. It governs vision, power and expansiveness. It is associated with the colour yellow.

- The heart chakra is located at the heart. It governs the sense of touch, compassion and love. It is associated with the colours green, or rose pink.
- The throat chakra is located at the throat. It controls the mouth and skin, the auditory sense and communication. It is connected to positive and negative attitudes to life. It is associated with the colour blue.
- The 'third eye' chakra is located slightly above and between the eyebrows. It governs our mental sense as well as our ability to trust. It is also the seat of wisdom and the connecting point between ourselves and the universal consciousness. It is associated with the colour indigo.
- The crown chakra is located at the top of the head. It is said to be all-transcending. From here we have the ability to connect with a higher consciousness. It is associated with the colours gold, violet or white

Working with the chakras is a potent way of ensuring body, mind and soul are always in harmony.

Getting Physical – Doing the Postures

Getting started

It is not easy keeping to any practice routine at home. But it may be easier than dragging yourself out to a class on cold winter nights. However, you do have to practise. It is the only way you will benefit. Regular and consistent work pays off. Even if you go to classes, it pays to supplement what you do there with some daily practice.

The good news is that you do not have to do that much. Not everyone is dedicated enough to get up at the crack of dawn every day to practise. Try and make your yoga practice work for you, so it becomes something you enjoy. Do it with a friend or in office lunch hours, or make it part of your routine when you get back from work.

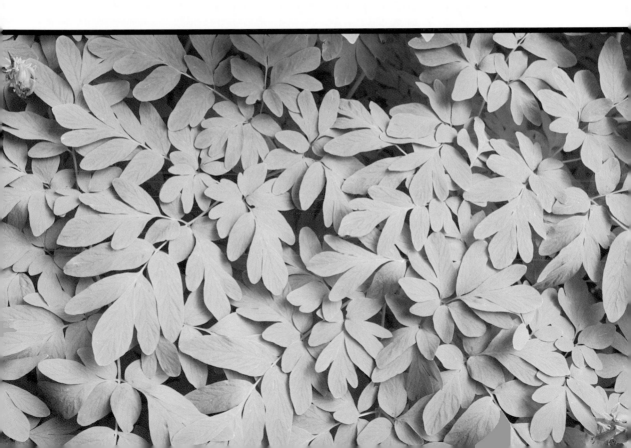

When to practise

There are ten exercises listed here – that's a short routine, which you should be able to fit into the day. The whole session should not take longer than 45 minutes. You will take more time at first, while you are learning. In time you will find you feel 'not quite right' on the days you don't practise. Your body will start to need yoga!

You can divide the practice up into separate times during the day. Maybe do the warming up and the cat pose first thing in the morning; the four standing postures at midday; the sitting postures late afternoon; and the spinal twist and the shoulderstand before going to bed. That makes ten to fifteen minutes a session – which should be achievable! If you decide to practise in separate sessions, begin each one with a short relaxation, breathing and warming up exercises.

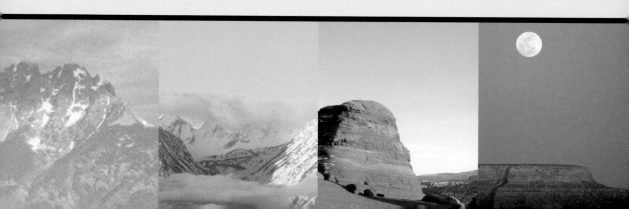

Before you start

There are certain practical things to bear in mind:

- If you have a medical condition, you should only train with a properly qualified yoga teacher, and consult your doctor first.
- If you are pregnant, do not start a yoga programme as a beginner. Consult a yoga teacher and only continue if you know what you are doing.
- During menstruation, listen to your body. You may need to rest completely from yoga postures for the first couple of days. Do not do any inverted postures during your period.
- Do not eat beforehand – three hours for a meal, two hours for a snack.
- If possible, have bowels and bladder empty.
- Wear loose clothing that you can move freely in.
- Feet should be bare. The floor can be carpeted but make sure you can have a firm grip – no deep shag pile. On bare floors, practise the sitting and lying postures on a non-slip mat.
- Make sure the practice room is warm and that you are unlikely to cool down – have spare clothing to hand if necessary.

First – relax!

All yoga sessions should start with a brief relaxation. Lie on the floor, stretch your arms and feet out to the sides. Wriggle your back around on the floor, easing any tension. Now bend your knees, with feet on the floor close to the buttocks. Take the back of the head in the hands, lift it slightly and ease out the back of the neck. Make sure the back of the neck stays slightly elongated as you replace your head on the floor, with the chin tucked slightly downwards. Replace the arms on the floor, at a 45 degree angle from the sides of your body, the palms of your hands facing upwards. Feel as if your whole spine is dropping towards the floor. Feel the contact of all the vertebrae with the floor.

Now stretch your legs out along the floor. As you inhale, gently contract and release each area of the body, relaxing as you exhale. Start with the feet, continue to the legs, buttocks, waist, torso, shoulders, arms, hands and fingers. Then the face. When you have finished, mentally check your whole body. See if anywhere still feels tense. Areas that hold tensions that are often hard to shift are the face, shoulders and stomach.

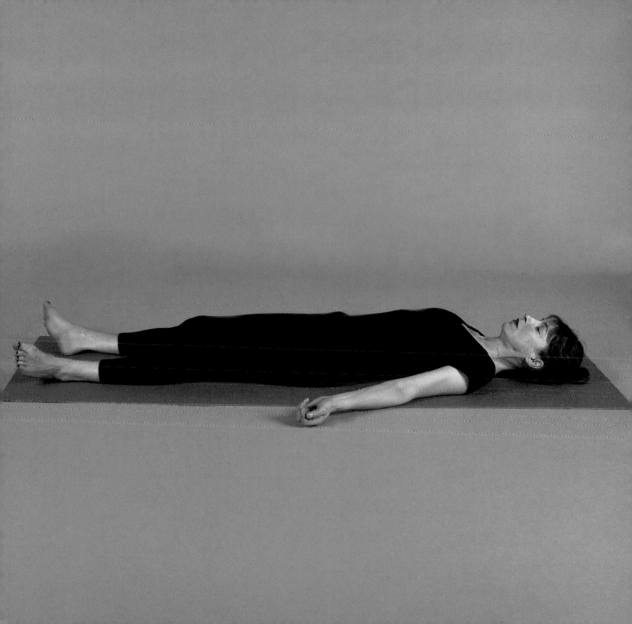

Deep breathing

Now you are ready to breathe. The essence of yogic breathing is very simple: it's just breathing completely, as you did when you were a small baby. Watch children or animals as they sleep – you will see exactly what deep, rhythmic breathing is. Now you can relearn it.

First stretch your whole body deeply. Extend from the waist: upwards with torso, arms and hands; downwards with belly, buttocks, legs and feet. Bend your knees with your feet close to the buttocks and place the palms of your hands over the bottom of the rib cage. The middle fingers should be just touching, an inch or two above the navel. Become aware of how you breathe normally. Are you using only part of your lungs? Is only your upper chest moving? Our breathing patterns are closely connected to our emotions – so tune in to how you are feeling, and how your feelings change as your breathing pattern changes.

Now breathe in, feeling the rib cage expanding. Try to fill the bottom portion of the lungs first, allowing them to swell towards the top. Then as you exhale, deflate the lungs from the top down. Feel the movement of the abdomen, with the fingers gently moving away from one another on the in-breath. Continue with this rhythmic rising and falling, allowing the breath to feel easy and unrestricted. In particular, do not try to breathe in or breathe deeply. Concentrate instead on the exhalation, allowing it to be as complete as possible, and the in-breath will come of its own accord. Trying to 'do' deep breathing will only result in strain. Do this for ten inhalations and exhalations. Then return to natural, normal, relaxed breathing. Stretch out again.

When you are doing the postures never hold your breath, but breathe as normally as you can. Imagine yourself taking in energy with the in-breath, and allowing that energy to circulate around the body. Allow the breath to come and go, without letting it become tense, even when the posture seems difficult.

Warming up exercises

Always warm and limber your body before you start the proper exercises. Make sure you are on a carpet or thick mat, or even a folded blanket. After breathing and stretching out, wriggle your body around on the floor. Press the back down, and the small of the back, trying to remove the hollow. With your knees bent, raise your bottom off the floor, keeping the back of the neck as flat as you can. Now curl the spine back down on the floor, starting with the top and pressing each vertebra down one by one until the small of the back is resting on the floor. Repeat twice.

Now bring the knees into the chest, hugging them with your hands and keeping the back of the head on the floor. Start to rock gently backwards and forwards on the floor, with the back rounded, this time lifting your head as you rock forwards, while trying to lift your bottom off the floor and roll onto your shoulders as you rock back. As you rock, feel as if you are massaging the spine. Now try and speed up the momentum until you come to a standing position – preferably without using your hands!

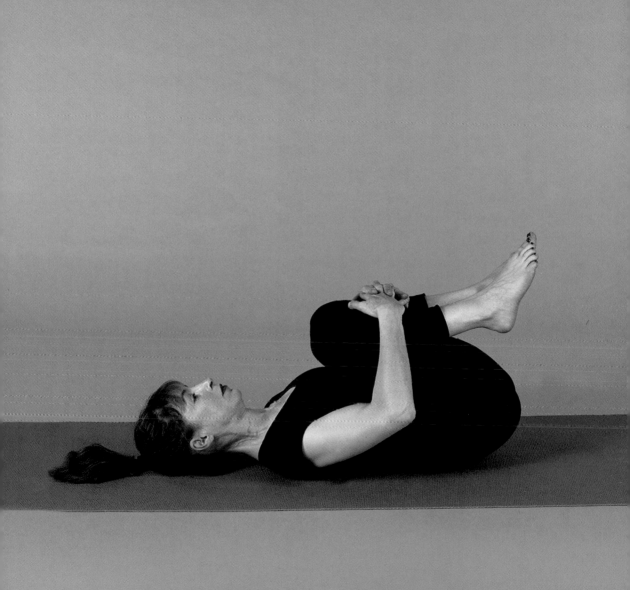

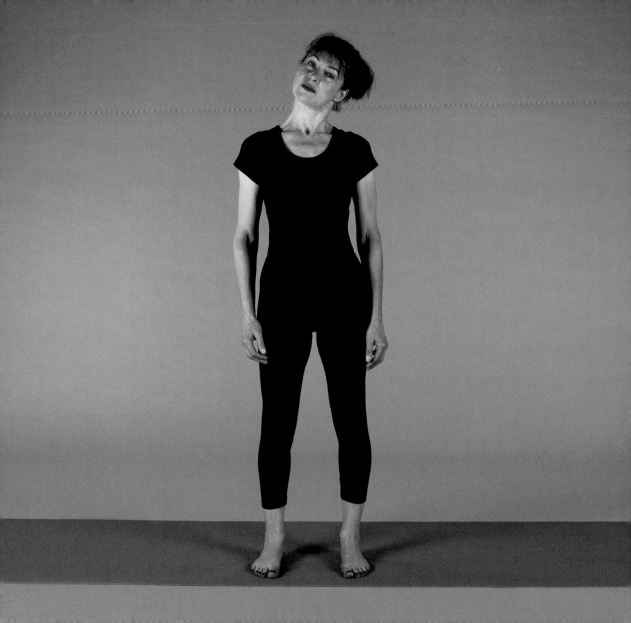

As you come to your feet, bend forwards from the waist and hang with the feet about a hip's width apart. Allow yourself to feel loose and floppy. Let the back of the neck relax and the tension ease out of the shoulders. Move the shoulders and the torso around a little and let the head hang – this is not a rigid position. Keep the arms and hands released. Now come up gradually. Uncurl the spine, as if you are resting one vertebra on top of the other. Keep the arms and hands relaxed. Let the head stay relaxed and bring it up last of all.

Now begin to limber the whole body. Gently move the head from one side to the other as if you want each ear to touch the shoulder. Feel the muscles stretching on either side of the neck. Move slowly and carefully three times to each side. Gently allow the head to fall back, opening the mouth. Bring the head back to the centre, then let it come forwards, with the chin towards the chest. Do this three times, finally bringing the head upright and facing forwards.

Now raise both shoulders to the ears, relaxing them as they fall. Do this three times. Next shake out each arm, giving it a really good shake until you feel the blood circulating fully and the hands becoming warm. Then, with feet further apart, swing your body round from the waist, with your arms and head following the movement round. Bend your knees each time you swing to the back. Feel the body getting warmer. Make six swings to each side. Then shake out each leg, and each foot, until they feel very loose and floppy.

Finally, stand once more with your feet hip-width apart, feet parallel and toes pointing forwards, and close your eyes. Place the weight firmly over both feet, resting neither on the ball of the foot nor the heels. Allow the legs to be firm and feel solid, with the kneecaps lightly drawn up. Feel as if you are creating space around the midriff; that is, between the lower rib cage and the hips. Allow the spine to feel relaxed but erect and let the shoulders, arms and hands relax. Lengthen the neck lightly, and keep the underneath of the chin parallel to the floor. Imagine you have a string coming from the top of your head, attached to the ceiling. Stand with the eyes gently closed, try to feel light, yet solid and firm; breathe evenly and regularly. Enjoy the feeling of strength, solidity and balance.

Now open your eyes, relax your knees, stretch your hands upwards on an inhalation, and exhale through your mouth as you allow the whole body to flop forwards from the waist, bending your knees as you do so. (But be careful — If you have any trouble with the lower back, do not do this exercise.)

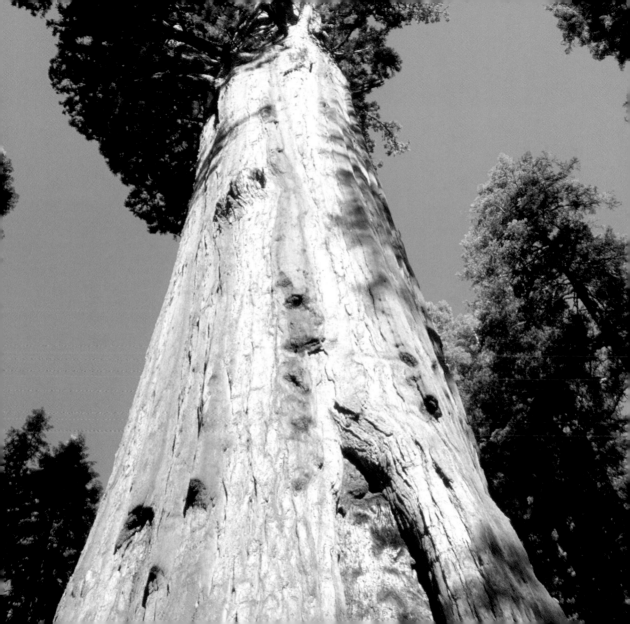

Cat pose

The cat pose is the final stage of your warming up session. Go down on all fours, with your hands on the floor directly underneath your shoulders, fingers straight out in front of you. Your knees are on the floor with the thighs at right-angles to the floor, the tops of the feet stretched out behind you. Take two even breaths in this position. On the next inhalation, raise the head as if you are looking up and hollow your back (see photo p.44). Try not to tense your shoulders. As you exhale, bring your head in, moving the chin towards the chest, and make your back round, bringing the belly up.

Repeat these movements, breathing evenly. Try as you move to concentrate your mind fully on the body, gradually extending the range of movement in the spine. Be aware of any places that feel rigid or stiff – it is normal for some parts of the spine to move more flexibly than others. Work on getting more movement into these stiff places rather than over-extending the places that are already flexible. Continue with the cat pose for six inhalations and exhalations.

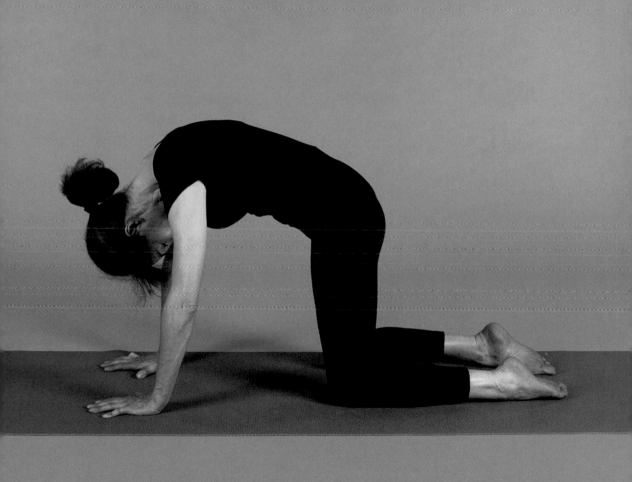

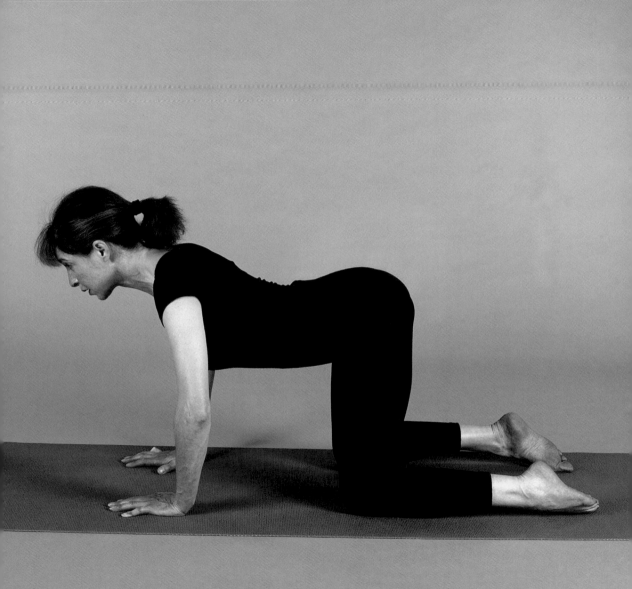

Finish by sitting back with your bottom on your heels, forehead on the floor, and the arms stretched out in front of you with palms facing down and forwards, elbows as straight as possible. Now clasp your hands behind the base of the spine, and gently ease yourself onto the top of your head, raising your bottom off the floor and straightening your arms, raising the hands out behind you with the elbows straight. Do this three times, sitting back onto the heels in between the stretches. Finally, relax with your bottom back on your heels, forehead on the floor, and your arms resting by the side of your feet with the palms facing up. If you want to do a quick warm-up just do the cat pose, followed by this raised-arm stretch.

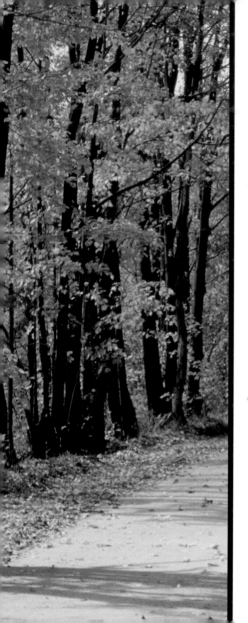

Points to remember

- As you undergo the postures, try to make them exercises in concentration at the same time. Tune into your body: what you are feeling, where you are stuck, where you move easily. Try not to allow your mind to wander. Of course it will, but become aware that this is happening and bring yourself back into a full involvement with what you are doing.

- Be aware of your mental attitude to the practice – whether you try too hard; whether you give up too soon; whether you are put into a negative frame of mind because of the difficulties; whether you see them as challenging or overwhelming.

- Each practice will be different – your body may be sluggish or responsive, your mind fresh or burdened. Simply be aware of all this, without judging it. Physically, the exercises should certainly provide you with a stretch, but do stop at any sign of strain.

- The more you can relax into the posture, pushing just so much but not enough to create new stresses, the better your practice will become. Yoga is always about finding balance.

- The time you spend holding a posture will vary according to your own fitness and needs. If you are a complete beginner and not very fit, hold each posture for just one breath. As you become stronger and more adept, increase the number of breaths you take to a maximum of five.

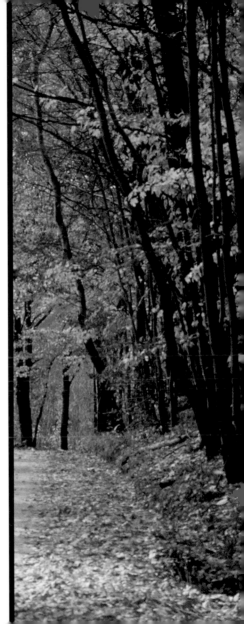

Standing postures

(Sanskrit names are in brackets)

Triangle

(Utthita trikonasana)

This is your first classic yoga posture. Stand with your feet two to three feet apart; the exact distance will depend on your personal body proportions. Long-legged people will require more space; shorter people less. Stand so you feel well-balanced and supported. Now turn your right foot sideways so the toes point towards the right and turn the left foot slightly inwards so that the left instep is in line with the right heel. Place your hands on your hips and turn the torso to face forwards. You will probably feel awkward in this position at first – don't worry. Try to keep the knees straight and the legs strong. Feel the space around the midriff by drawing the torso upwards while standing firmly. Try to avoid hollowing the base of the spine.

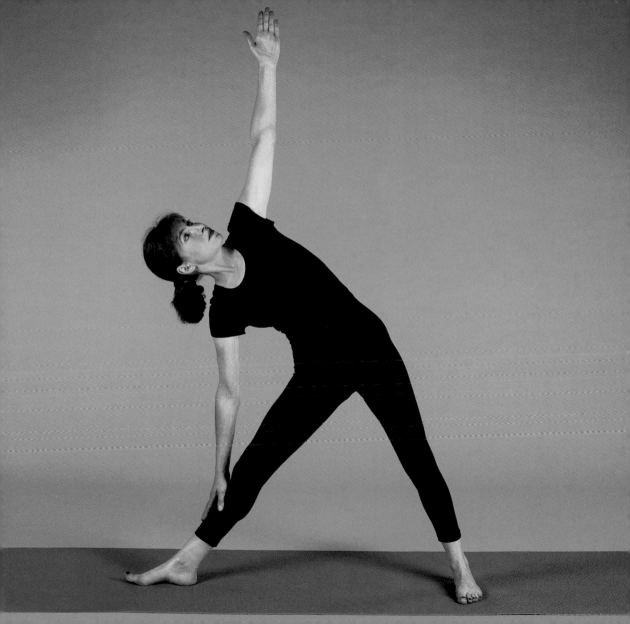

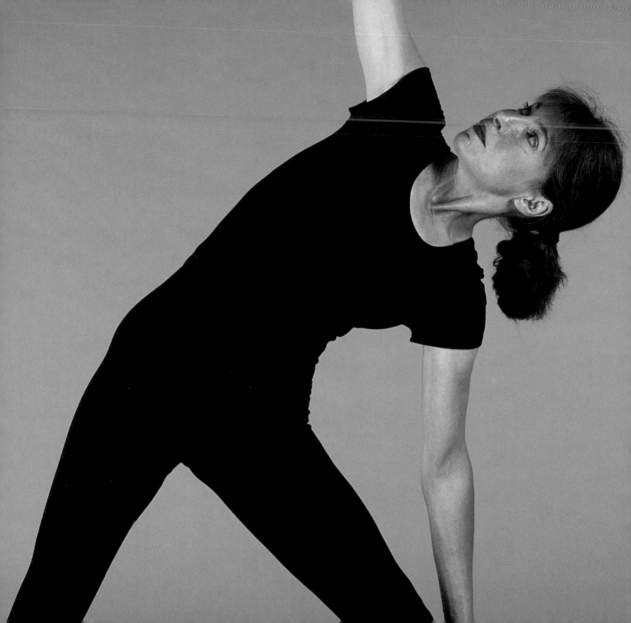

Now lift the arms gently sideways to shoulder level, stretching them so they are parallel to the floor with the fingers straight. Keep the shoulders down and, as far as possible, relaxed. Now gently lower the right hand so it comes to the side of the right thigh, and the whole of the left side is gently stretched. Then raise the left arm vertically, with the palm facing forwards and the fingers pointing directly towards the ceiling.

Keeping the legs straight, guide the right hand as far down the right leg as it will stretch, holding the left arm upwards and the left hip facing upwards rather than caving in towards the front. Then slowly and gently move up, and move both arms back into the sideways stretched position. Lower the arms and turn the feet so the toes are facing forwards.

Shake the body out gently, from the feet to the shoulders and the face. Be aware of any tensions and relax them out. Then perform the triangle posture to the other side; that is, with the left foot facing leftwards and the right turned in at a left angle. The arms come out to the sides, then the left hand goes down the left leg, the right is upstretched. Come out of the pose as before and shake out any tensions.

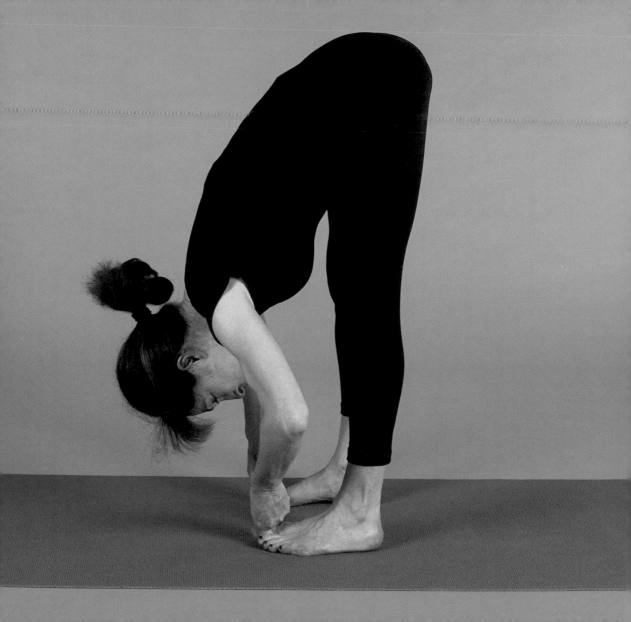

Head to knee

(Uttanasana)

Stand with your feet about hip-width apart, feet facing forwards and parallel to each other. Now bend forwards from the waist, and take the hands towards the floor, as far down as is possible without straining, keeping the knees lifted and the legs straight. Catch hold of the ankles if you can; if not, place the hands behind the calves or knees. Now, keeping the legs straight, gently draw the torso down and inwards towards the legs. Think in terms of taking the stomach towards the thighs rather than lowering the head towards the knees. In this way, the spine will lengthen and stretch. Keep the shoulders, back of the neck and the face relaxed, and keep the weight evenly centred over both feet. Try to relax the base of the spine.

To come out of the posture, relax the knees, arms and hands and, staying in the bent position, shake the body around loosely. Now draw up the kneecaps again, and raise the torso gradually, with the head coming up last, as described in the 'Warming Up' section (*see page* 30).

Wide leg stretch

(Prasarita padottanasana)

Stand with the legs between four and five feet apart, the toes pointing forwards. Draw the kneecaps up and straighten the legs, using the thigh muscles. Ensure your weight is evenly placed over both feet. Now lean forwards and place your hands on the floor in front of you, with the palms flat on the floor and the fingers pointing forwards. Then gradually walk the hands inwards as far as you can; ideally they will be in line with the feet, but as near that position as is possible for you will do. Do not sacrifice the knee and leg position!

To come out of the posture, allow the knees to relax slightly and walk the hands forwards. Shift the feet closer together until they are hip-width apart, then shake the body loosely to relax it. Draw up the kneecaps once more and gently raise the torso as before, gradually building the vertebrae up, one on top of the other, with the shoulders and head, relaxed and hanging, coming up last.

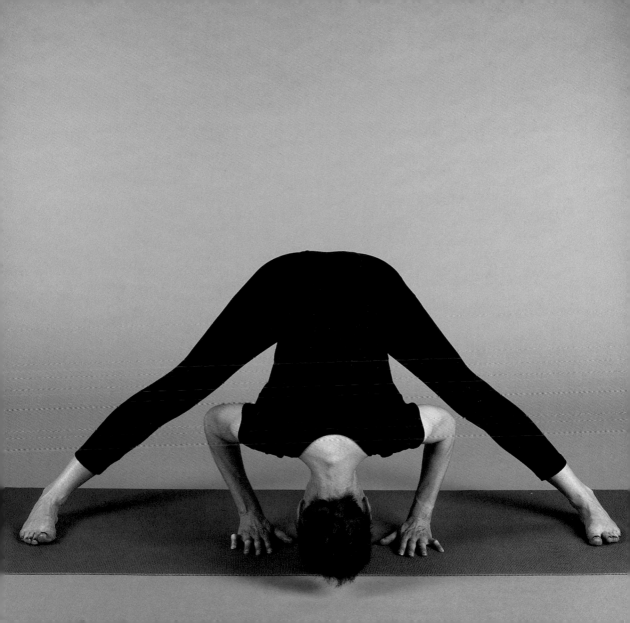

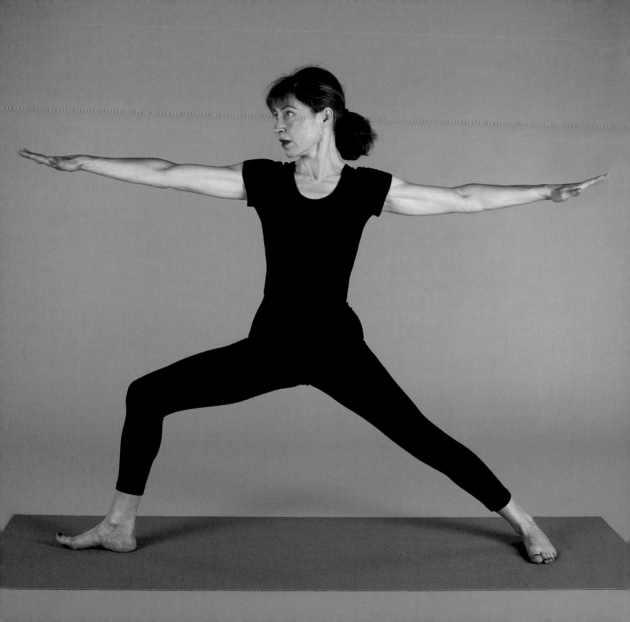

Warrior

(Virabhadrasana)

Stand with your feet four to five feet apart. Turn the right foot out so it faces towards the right, and the left in so it is facing the same direction, as in the triangle (*see page* 42). Turn the torso forwards, keeping the feet in position. Raise the arms sideways so they are parallel to the floor, with fingers extended and palms facing downwards.

Bend the right knee and lower the right thigh. Ideally the thigh should move so it is parallel to the floor, but try at the same time to keep the left leg as straight as possible. Look to the right, over the right fingertips. Keep the torso upright, the back straight and the arms up. The right knee should be kept above the right foot rather than caving in towards the front. Keep the shoulders down and relaxed. Keep breathing! To release the posture, raise the right knee and straighten the right leg, face the front, lower the arms, relax the legs, move the feet closer to one another and shake out any tensions.

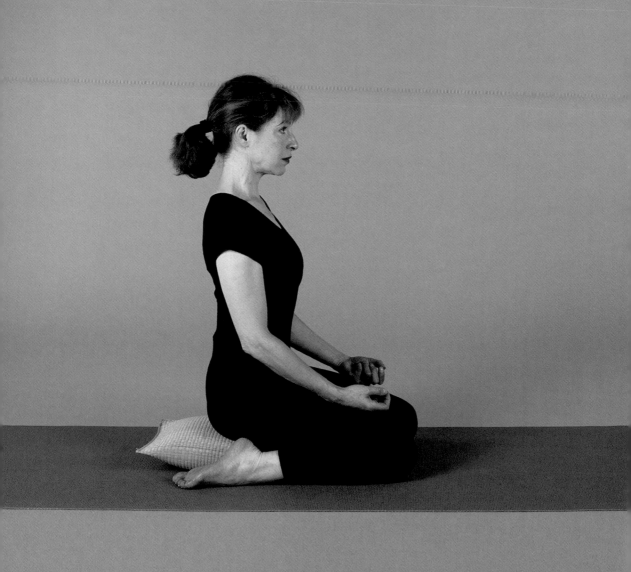

Sitting and lying postures
Hero pose (Virasana)

Sit on your heels, with the knees bent and close together, the front of
the feet down against the floor, toes pointing back. Now, if you can,
move the heels apart, still with the feet in position rather than splaying
out, and try to sit on the floor between the heels, keeping the knees as
close together as possible. If this is impossible (which it may well be at
first, due to tight ankles or legs), you can place a pile of books or a firm
cushion under your buttocks, between the feet. Don't make it too easy
– the posture should gradually ease and stretch the legs and ankles.

Try in the posture to keep the small of the back extended and flat
rather than caving in, and to draw the spine up, keeping the shoulders
and the back of the neck relaxed. The hands can rest in your lap or at
the sides. The face should be relaxed and looking forwards, with the
chin parallel to the floor. To come out of the posture, ease yourself
back up to sit on the heels, then release the legs so they are straight in
front of you, and shake them out loosely to relax any tension.

Cobbler pose

(Baddha konasana)

Sit with your buttocks on the floor and your knees bent out to the sides, the soles of the feet together and the heels as close in towards the perineum as possible. Clasp your hands around the feet, and draw the spine up, keeping the base of the spine flat. Now gently attempt to open the feet out, so the inside edges of the feet move further apart, the outside edges pressing together.

As you make this movement, the knees should descend as far as possible towards the floor. Make sure you keep the back extended, and the shoulders down and relaxed.
To come out of the posture, release the back and hands and allow the knees to raise. Make your back round, clasp the arms loosely around the legs, and drop the head lightly between the knees. Shake out any tension.

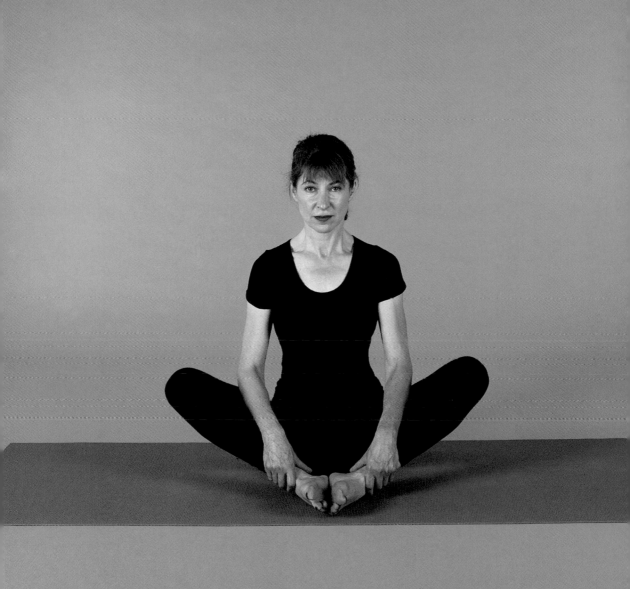

Forward bend

(Pascimottanasana)

Sit in an L-shape, with your legs out in front of you, your toes facing upwards. If you like, you can prop yourself up lightly with your hands placed on the floor at your sides. Try to sit up on your 'sitting bones', that is, the underside of the pelvis. Ensure the spine is straight, with the lower ribs extending away from the hip bones and creating space around the midriff. Keep the shoulders and face relaxed.

Now extend the hands down the legs as far as you can, without sacrificing the straight position of the legs. Ideally, the hands should be placed around the feet, or the index finger around the big toe. If you cannot manage this, it may help to have a tie, soft belt or thin scarf to hand, which you can hook around the feet, holding onto each end with the hands. Whether using the tie or your hands, the idea is to lever your torso gradually downwards over the legs.

As with the head to knee pose, think in terms of the stomach coming towards the thighs and the spine gently elongating, as if you are

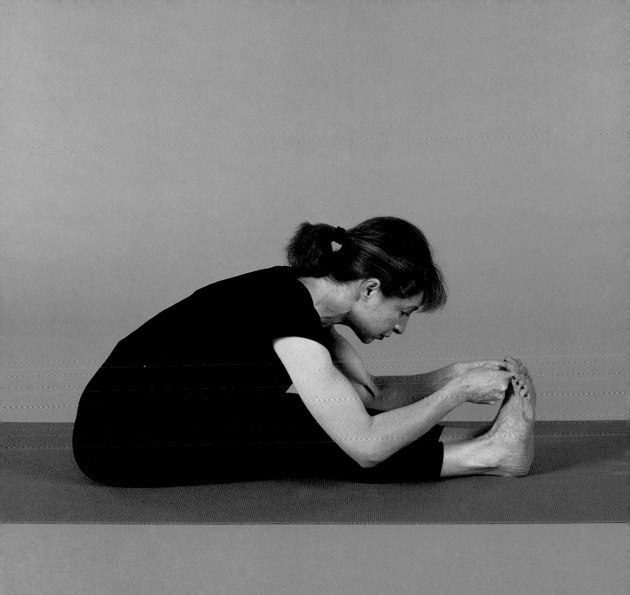

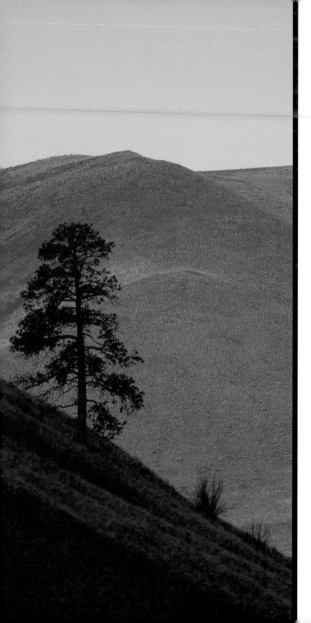

making a hairpin shape. Do not
drop the head towards the legs
and let the back become round!
Make sure all the time that the
back of the knees are pressing
down towards the floor, and the
legs stay straight. Do not pull
with the arms and shoulders.
Breathe quietly and normally.
Continue easing yourself down
gently, visualizing the spine
lengthening like a piece of elastic.
To come out of the posture,
release the hands or the tie, bend
the knees slightly, and allow the
torso to flop forwards. Shake out
any tensions and wriggle the
legs around.

Cobra

(Bhujangasana)

Lie front down on the floor, arms bent, palms down in front of you on the floor with the forehead on the back of the top hand. Allow the toes to face inwards and the heels to flop apart. Release any tensions, particularly from the lower back. Then place the hands underneath the shoulders, with the palms flat and the fingers facing forwards. The fingertips should be in line with the top of the shoulders, the elbows sticking out. Point the toes down so the soles of the feet are facing upwards.

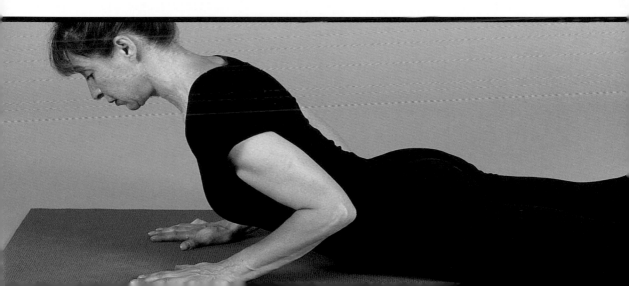

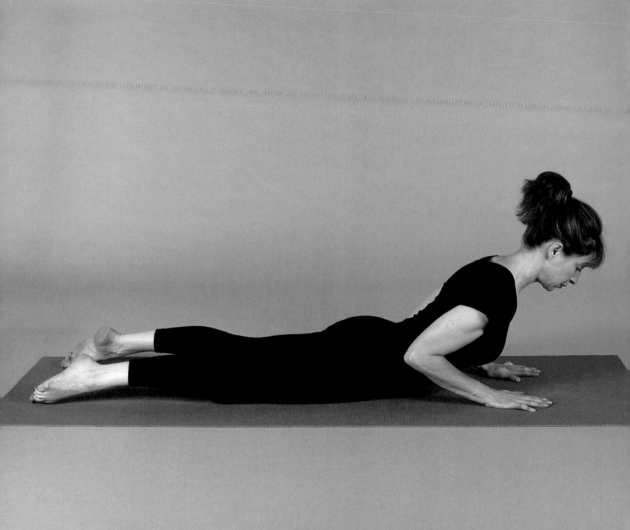

Now gently raise the torso off the floor. Try not to rely on the hands and arms, although you may press lightly down on the palms. Keep the shoulders relaxed and the face looking down towards the floor. As you raise the top part of the body from the floor, concentrate on extending the spine and using the muscles of the back to do the lifting. Press the hips gently into the floor to give you more support. Continue to breathe lightly and as normally as possible. Avoid the temptation to strain the lower back or tense the shoulders. Do not worry if you can hardly raise the body. This exercise improves the strength of the back and this will come in time.

To come out of the posture, gently lower the torso back to the floor, bend the arms in front of you again and rest one cheek on the back of the hands. Then go into the posture again, trying to lift a little further. Then lower the torso again, rest the other cheek on the back of the hands, release the feet and release any tension from the back.

Twisting posture

Spinal twist

(Bharadvajasana)

Sit on the floor and bend the left leg so the left foot turns inwards towards the right thigh, and your weight is slightly over onto the left buttock. Now bend the right leg, placing the right foot over the left thigh onto the floor. If you are unable to do this comfortably, you may extend the left leg and simply place the right foot flat on the floor outside the extended left knee.

Now try as far as you can to sit evenly on both buttocks, and to extend the spine. As in previous postures, feel as if the midriff is lengthening and the torso is lifting up out of the pelvis – try not to collapse in the middle. Place the palm of the left hand behind you on the floor by the buttocks. Using this hand as a lever, try to extend the spine a little more. Drop the right buttock by releasing any tension. Now straighten the right arm across the body, with the right elbow pushing against the

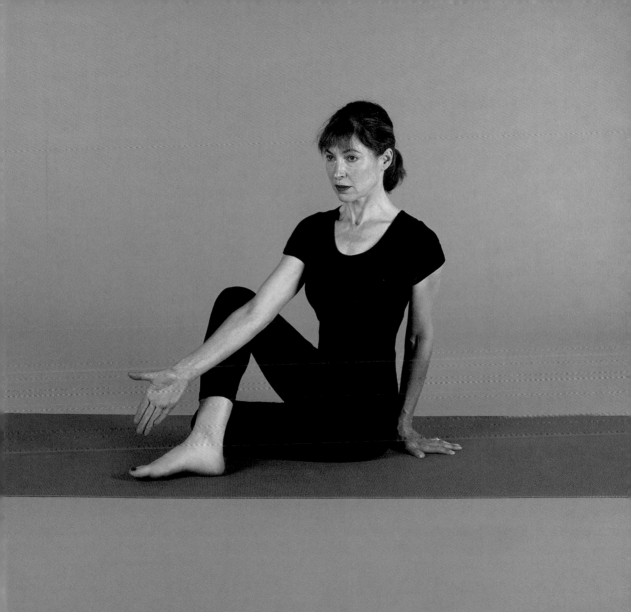

inside of the right knee and the right palm stretched outwards towards the left. Using this right arm as a lever, turn the whole torso leftwards from the waist. Make sure you are keeping the spine long and upright. Resist any temptation to twist the neck and head to the left. Simply keep the head in line with the torso, and turn the whole body from the waist, pressing down all the time with the right buttock. Try not to put tension into the shoulders. Breathe lightly and evenly.

To come out of the posture, release the arms, turn the torso back to the front, untwist the legs and shake them out in front of you. Then repeat the posture to the other side, with the right leg bent inwards, the left foot on the floor outside the right knee, the right hand behind you and the left arm coming across the body with its elbow levering against the inside of the left knee. Turn the whole body from the waist towards the right. Release, and shake out any tension as before.

Inverted posture

Shoulderstand

(Salamba sarvangasana)

Women should not perform this posture during the first days of menstruation. Lie on the floor on your back with your knees bent. Lift the head in the palms of the hands to ease the back of the neck out gently. Replace the head on the floor, making sure the back of the neck is stretched and the chin pointing downwards towards the chest. Place your hands by your sides. Now take the feet off the floor, and try to extend your legs backwards over your face, lifting your buttocks from the floor and rolling onto your upper back. You may support the buttocks or the small of the back with the hands. Gently ease yourself as far as you can onto the shoulders, gradually supporting yourself with your hands further and further up the back towards the shoulders. You may feel some constriction in your upper chest or throat. This should clear as you get more used to the posture.

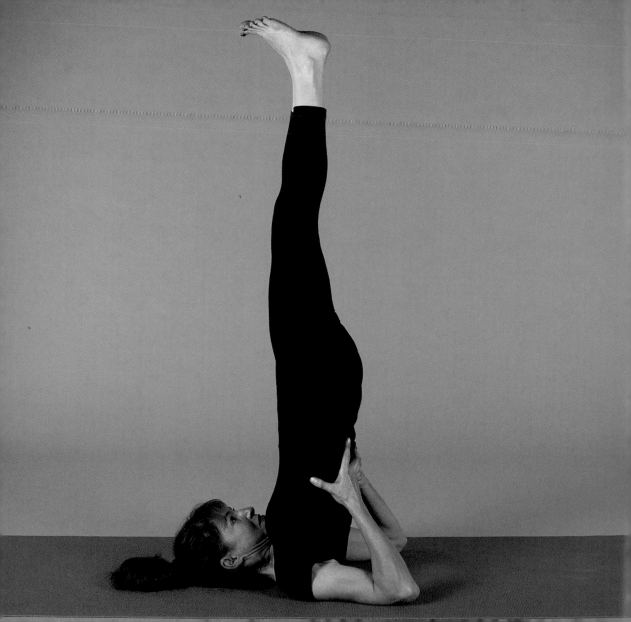

As you become more sure of your balance on your shoulders, you may attempt to lift the legs. The important thing is to make sure the back is extended and straight before bringing the legs up in the air. Ultimately there should be a straight line from the feet to the shoulders, with the underside of the feet uppermost and the toes relaxed and pointing backwards. Try all the time to work the hands further up the back in the direction of the shoulders, bringing the elbows closer together. There should be minimum pressure on the upper back and shoulders – the weight should be distributed evenly throughout the body.

To come out of the posture, drop the tips of the toes back beyond the top of the head, touching the floor if possible and rounding the back gently. Now slide the legs forwards, keeping them bent, with the knees close to the face, and the hands loosely stretched beyond the top of the head. Keep the knees bent, feet in the air, and push the back of the waist down into the floor to relieve any pressure. Place the feet on the floor and keeping the back of the neck extended, clasp the bent knees into the chest, then release the legs and slide them out along the floor with the toes relaxing outwards.

Finishing a session –

Breathing exercises

We can live for weeks without food, for days without water, yet without breathing we would be dead in minutes. Breath is quite simply our connection to life.

Breathing exercises have many functions. They can help us get more oxygen, and dispel carbon dioxide more effectively. They can make us feel more invigorated and keep our whole system working more effectively. And, since breathing is also intimately bound up with our nervous system, conscious control of the breath process can alter our emotional state and be a step towards meditative practices.

The following are the simplest yoga breathing practices. They can be carried out at the end of a session, before deep relaxation. You should sit down comfortably to do them, either on the floor (on a cushion or blanket if you prefer) with legs folded, or sitting in a chair that does not allow you to go to sleep!

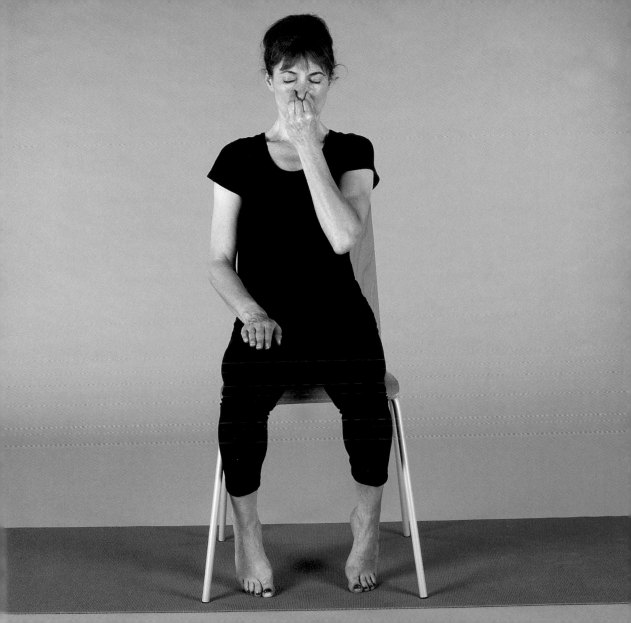

Alternate nostril breathing

(Anuloma viloma)

Press the right thumb against the right nostril to close it gently. Breathe in through the left nostril. Bring the ring finger to the left nostril and close it too, holding the breath briefly, then release the right nostril and breathe out slowly and evenly through it while keeping the left closed. Breathe in through the right, still keeping the left nostril closed, then close both nostrils briefly before releasing the left nostril and exhaling through it.

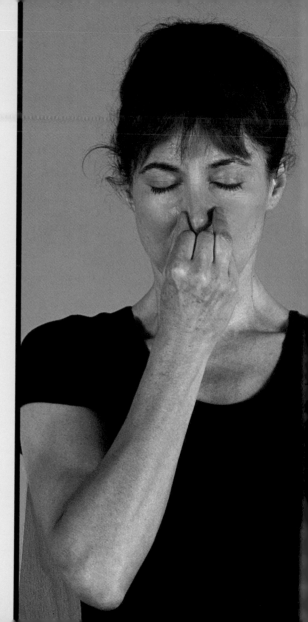

Repeat this series six times. The exercise should have a calming, harmonizing effect; do it whenever you are feeling stressed and unquiet.

Head-clearing exercise

(Kapalabhati)

This is a rather forceful exercise, which has exactly the described effect. Breathe out completely through the nose and pull the abdominal area well in. As you inhale, let the abdomen relax out. Do this quickly (about two breaths per second), for up to 20 breaths, ensuring in particular that each exhalation is strong and forceful.

Deep
relaxation

The best way to use this relaxation session is to read it through thoroughly so you become very familiar with it. Then make a tape of the instructions, giving yourself enough time to carry each one out. You may also like to practise it in turns with a friend, one reading the instructions to the other. Make sure that you have something soft to lie on, although it should not be so soft that you go to sleep immediately. Often we go to sleep still full of muscular tension, as well as with our minds still churning away. This is a slow, guided process of letting go with 'awareness'. If you do sleep afterwards it will be a deeply rewarding rest.

Lie on the floor with your knees bent, your feet on the floor and your arms resting loosely on the floor beyond the top of your head. Close your eyes gently. Take a few easy breaths. Now let the legs drop until they are fully extended on the floor. Lie with the feet two to three foot apart, the toes dropping outwards. If you have any back problems you can keep the knees bent. Bring the arms down so that they are lying at

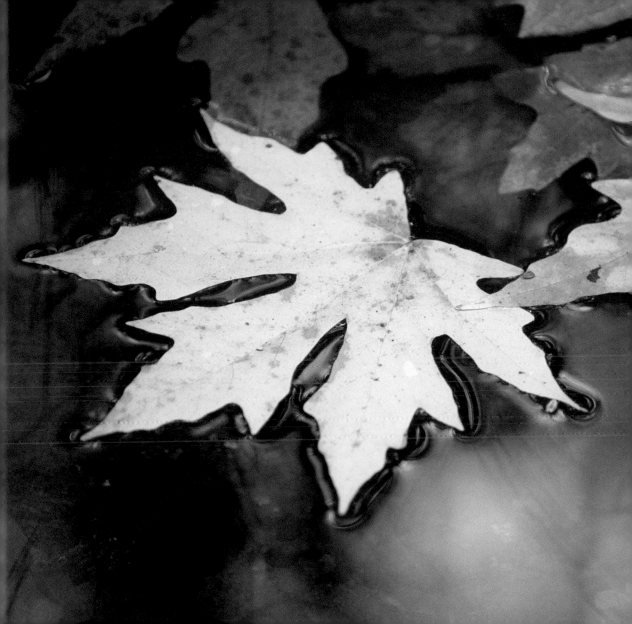

a 45-degree angle from the sides of the body, the palms facing upwards. Make sure the back of the neck is extended and that the back of the head is resting on the floor. Bring yourself into the 'here and now'. Drop any thoughts of what you have been doing, what you are going to do. Be aware of any sounds around you, from the street or garden outside, or from indoors. Become aware of what you are lying on, the feeling of the rug or carpet, the temperature of the air, the pulsation of your circulation, the rhythm of your heart.

Become aware of your toes. Wriggle them gently, contract them, then let them go. As you let go, feel any tension draining away from them and allow them to feel soft and heavy. Now bring your attention into the feet, contract them slightly then let go, feeling any tension draining away. Let the feeling of relaxation continue up into the ankles, allowing them to feel soft and heavy. Then bring the relaxation up into the legs. Feel the points where your body is in contact with the floor – the calves, the weight of the back of the thighs. Feel those contact points becoming heavier, feel any tension points easing and releasing. Allow yourself to become aware of the heaviness of the legs, of their weight on the floor. Now feel the buttocks resting on the floor. Feel any tension seeping out of the body. Feel the whole of the area around the pelvis relax, allow yourself to let go in the hips, deep into the lower abdomen. Allow the whole abdominal area to relax. Allow this relaxed feeling to rise up into the waist, all around the waist into the small of the back.

Now feel the sides of the torso relaxing. Feel as if the body is gently expanding, with its sides dropping further apart from each other. Feel the skin soften, the diaphragm and stomach loosen. Let the rib cage gently expand, let the movement of the lungs and heart become slow and relaxed. Feel the relaxation deep in the chest; as you breathe out let the chest feel freer and softer. Allow the whole of the back to relax. Feel each contact point as it lays on the floor; at each of these points feel the body soften and release. Allow this feeling of expanding and releasing to fill the

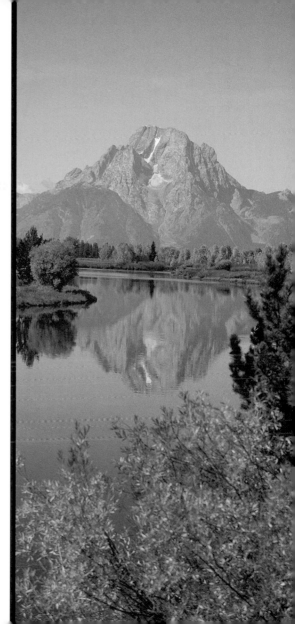

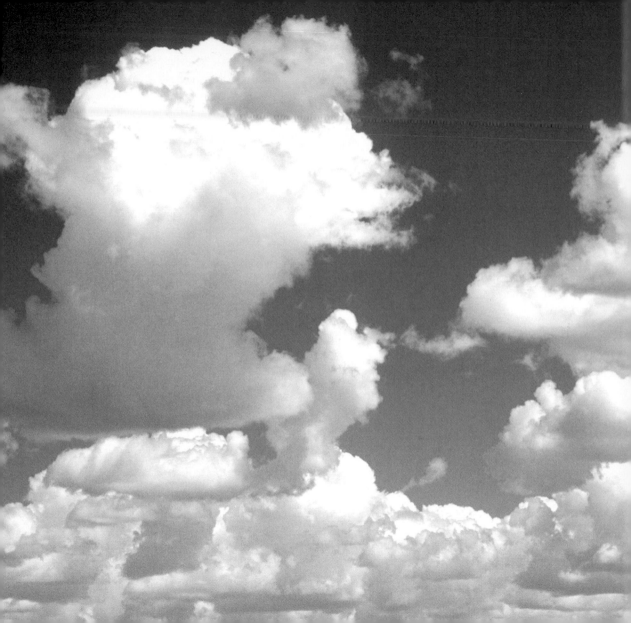

shoulders. Let any tension drain away, through the shoulders and the arms, out through the wrists and hands and fingers. Let the elbows relax, and the wrist joints; let the fingers gently curl. Feel the heaviness of the hands as they rest on the floor. Sigh out any remaining tension; on each out-breath imagine yourself becoming heavier and heavier.

Now feel the relaxation in your neck. Feel the softness of the skin on the neck and feel the top of the spine gently at rest. Allow this feeling of relaxation to travel all the way down the whole of the spine; trace the spine to the coccyx – the tailbone – just between the buttocks. Then travel in your imagination up the spine again, resting it even more heavily against the floor. Let the face relax. Allow the jaw to drop open slightly, the lips to part and feel soft. Let the tongue rest behind the lower teeth. Let the cheeks relax, feel the weight of the eyeballs resting gently back in the eye sockets. Feel the scalp loosen and relax. Feel the heavy weight of the head on the floor. Feel the easy, gentle flow of breath as it flows evenly through both nostrils. Trace the passage of the breath, down past the back of the throat, easily and gently into the lungs. Each time you breathe in, feel the whole body soften and expand. Each time you breathe out, feel yourself become more heavy and released. Allow everything to relax: skin, muscles, internal organs, nerves, bones.

Allow the mind to relax. Be aware of any thoughts, but simply watch them, noting their presence as if they are floating across the mind like clouds. Watch them come into the mind, see their shape and pattern, texture and colour. Then watch them gently slip away. Be aware of them but not affected by them. Savour this deep, relaxed state for as long as you please.

When you feel ready, start to deepen the in-breath. As you breathe in, begin to imagine you are taking fresh energy and life into the body. Still staying very relaxed, allow the energy to travel round the body, down to the toes, into the fingers, along the limbs. Feel the energy begin to move you, start to move the toes, then the fingers. Let the body come back to life, slowly bringing the feet together, stretching out. Allow yourself to stretch very gently, without disturbance. Bring the hands up beyond the top of the head, stretch all along the left side of the body, from the tips of the toes to the fingertips, then relax that side and stretch the right. Release again, and this time stretch diagonally, from the left toes up to the right fingertips. Release and reverse the stretch, from the left fingers to the right toes. Release and be aware of your gentle breathing. Keep the eyes closed.

Now curl the body over softly to the left side, like a foetus, and be aware of the beating of the heart. Then uncurl and sit up, with the eyes still closed, into a comfortable position, the spine upright and the head tilted forwards, chin towards the chest. Feel with each in-breath the energy returning to the spine and filling the whole body. Now place the palms of the hands over the eyes, open the eyes behind the hands, then take the hands away.

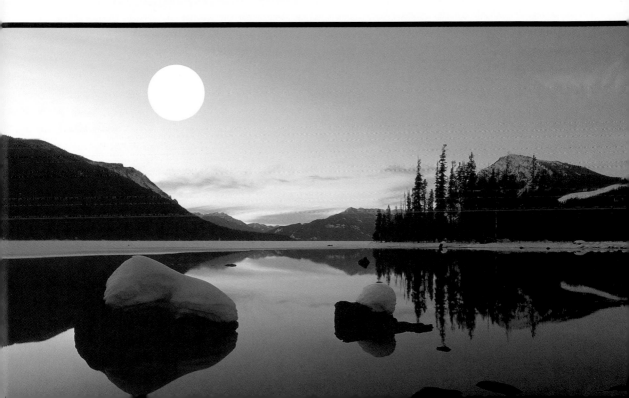

Yoga and Meditation

In our modern, stressed-out world peace seems to be one of the most sought after, hardest-to-find commodities. And this isn't a recent thing – life has always involved stress, or the sages of old would not have found ways of dealing with it. The ancient yogis had nothing less on their agenda than achieving transcendental bliss. But this isn't the main objective of people who turn to yoga today. Yoga provides practical ways in which we can all achieve greater peace amidst the daily strife.

Be here now

One way is to try to keep yourself 'here and now', totally involved and staying present in the moment. You can learn to do this through the practice of meditation. Meditation can change your world. Some people also believe that it can change the world. In ancient times, the reason for meditating was to arrive at supra-consciousness, a blissfully wide awake state. Nowadays meditation is a lifeline for many people, allowing them to see the mental disturbances of daily life for what they are – self-imposed barriers and stresses.

The Transcendental Meditation organization say that if enough people meditate at the same time, the consciousness of the planet will be raised, crime will disappear and there will be world peace.

In the meditative state you will feel 'in tune' with the universe and with your own being – maybe experience a loss of self; an 'aliveness' and a sense of deep connection. Your thoughts will feel stilled; not dull, but as if they are receding instead of interfering. Here is one of the more intense, powerful ways of experiencing the meditative state:

Meditation exercise

Sit in a relaxed, upright position. Check that the body is free of tension by contracting the muscles in each area from the feet up as you breathe in, then releasing all the muscles as you breathe out. Try to block out the external world and withdraw your senses as much as possible. Close your eyes and sit quietly. Imagine the loving presence of someone who cares or cared for you very deeply and unconditionally in the past. It may be a favourite aunt, a lover or a very good friend – someone who loved you exactly as you were. Try not to think of them as an individual, just allow yourself to sense their acceptance and support.

As you breathe in, fill yourself with this feeling. You may see it as colour, or light streaming into you. As you breathe out, let the feeling circulate all around your body. Feel it filling and expanding you, becoming part of you. If you have any particular area of pain or discomfort, allow the feeling to travel there and warm and release it. Now, as you breathe in, see the source of that love and feel as if you are growing so big that you can embrace and absorb it. Allow yourself and the feeling to become one and know that you are that pure self which was, is and always will be recognized and loved.

Yoga and Diet

It is now well-known that eating pure, cleansing foods – organic, wholemeal and largely vegetarian – rids the body of pollutants and increases its immunity to disease. What we often don't realize is the way in which we can purify our mental, spiritual and psychic systems as well. A yogic diet works in many ways. As the body becomes less burdened, thoughts become clearer and you will find yourself spiritually recharged. Cleaning up your life works on all levels!

Yoga practitioners have always avoided processed foods, living instead on simple food which is as fresh and close to its natural origins as possible. The further away food is from its source, the more contaminated it becomes. Food that has been treated scientifically to make it longer-lasting contains an increasing range of undesirable substances. As well as being unnecessary, these can often be harmful to our health and very addictive.

Following a yoga diet is another way of getting back to a state of natural balance. More and more it will become possible for you to assess for yourself the correct diet. Your enhanced sensitivity will help you know which foods to eat and which to avoid. Once you start to eat more simply it will become easier for you to distinguish the foods you need, and when you need them, instead of being confused by the unnatural combinations of prepackaged food.

The principles of the yoga diet are the basic ones known to anyone interested in health: mainly vegetarian and wholefood, with the emphasis on fresh, natural, unprocessed foods, simply prepared – vegetables, fruit, beans, wholegrains, nuts, seeds, and some dairy produce.

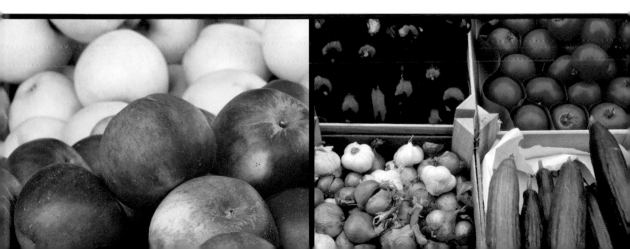

Yoga For Specific Problems

Yoga has answers for many common problems. Here, briefly, are some of them. If you have any long-term health problems, you are strongly recommended to contact a qualified yoga teacher for yoga therapy (*see Resource Guide*).

Asthma: Relaxation. Triangle. Cobra. Shoulderstand.
Deep breathing. Alternate nostril breathing.
Head-cleaning exercise.

Back pain: Forward bend. Deep relaxation.

Blood pressure (high): Forward bend. Shoulderstand.

Blood pressure (low): Hero pose. Shoulderstand (regulates blood flow).

Colds: Alternate nostril breathing.

Constipation: Head-cleaning exercise.

Depression: Cat pose. Deep breathing. Alternate nostril breathing. Head-cleaning exercise.

Diarrhoea: Relaxation. Shoulderstand.

Digestive problems: Cat pose. Cobra.

Headache: Slow warm-ups, including bending from the waist and slow uncurling to standing position. Starting session relaxation. Deep relaxation.

Painful periods: Cobbler pose. Forward bend. Cobra. Deep relaxation. Meditation.

Premenstrual tension; menopause: Cobbler pose.

Rheumatism and arthritis: Starting session warming up. Head-cleaning exercise.

Stress : Starting session relaxation. Starting session warming up. Cat pose. Deep relaxation Meditation.

Varicose veins: Shoulderstand.

Resource Guide

Astanga Vinyasa Yoga
12 Beatty Avenue
Coldean
Brighton
East Sussex BN1 9ED
Tel: 01273 687071

British Wheel of Yoga
1 Hamilton Place
Boston Road
Sleaford
Lincs NG34 7ES
Tel: 01529 306851

Himalayan International Institute
70 Claremont Road
London W13 0DG
Tel: 020 8991 8090

Iyengar Yoga
Maida Vale Yoga Institute
223a Randolph Avenue
London W9 1NL
Tel: 020 7624 3080

Sivananda Yoga Centre
51 Felsham Road
London SW15 1AZ
Tel: 020 8780 0160

Yoga Biomedical Trust
PO Box 140
Cambridge CB4 3SY
Tel: 01223 67301

Yoga Centre
Church Farm House
Spring Close Lane
Cheam
Surrey SM3 8PU
Tel: 020 8644 0309

Yoga for Health Foundation
Ickwell Bury
Northill
Near Biggleswade
Bedfordshire SG18 9EF
Tel: 01767 627271

**International Yoga Teachers'
Association**
c/o Shirley Deffert
15 Tarrow Close
Hornsby
2077 New South Wales
Australia

Ananda
14618 Tyler Foote Road
Nevada City
California 95959
USA
Tel: 916 292 3462

Omega Institute
260 Lake Drive
Rhinebeck
NY 12572
USA
Tel: 800 944 1001 or
914 266 4444

Unity and Yoga Association
4601 East Euclid Avenue
Phoenix
Arizona
USA